NATURAL FOLK REMEDIES

Work with Nature to Protect Your Body
and Promote Healing

Leroy D. Patterson

Table of Contents

CHAPTER 1 3

TURMERIC CHILI GINGER SHIITAKE EUCALYPTUS LAVENDER MINT FENUGREEK MAGNESIUM TAKEAWAY OVERVIEW YOU HAS PROBABLY TRIED A HOME REMEDY AT SOME POINT: 3

CHAPTER 2 25

TOP 6 BENEFITS OF TAKING COLLAGEN EVERYONE SHOULD BE AWARE OF THE FOLLOWING: 25

CHAPTER 3 31

BODY ODOR CAN BE REDUCED BY APPLYING BAKING SODA AND LEMON JUICE TO THE UNDERARMS. 31

THE END 41

CHAPTER 1

Herbal teas to treat cold, essential oils to ease a headache, and plant-based supplements to help you sleep better It could have been your grandmother or something you read online. The point is that you tried it, and now you might be wondering, "Should I try it again?"

What exactly makes a home remedy effective is unclear. Is it really a change in the body's physiological processes or more of a placebo effect? Fortunately, scientists have been asking the same questions in a lab over the past few decades, and they are discovering that some of our plant-based remedies are not just myths.

Therefore, we have your back for the skeptical individual who requires more than a placebo to feel well. The science-backed home remedies are as follows:

Turmeric for inflammation and pain who hasn't heard of it by now? For nearly 4,000 years, turmeric has been used in Ayurvedic medicine, mostly in South Asia. The golden spice may be most effective for relieving pain, particularly inflammation-related pain. This is due to its long list of documented medicinal uses.

Curcumin, according to a number of studies, is what gives turmeric its "wow" factor. In one study, people with arthritis pain found that taking 500 milligrams (mg) of curcumin reduced their pain levels more than 50 mg of an anti-inflammatory drug called diclofenac sodium.

This claim about pain relief is also supported by other studies, which found that treating knee osteoarthritis patients with pain with turmeric extract was just as effective as taking ibuprofen.

Avoid grinding turmeric because it has a strong odor! for, however, immediate relief. Because turmeric contains only 3% curcumin, it is preferable to take curcumin supplements for relief.

However, a calming turmeric latte will still be beneficial. A dose of 2 to 5 grams (g) of the spice may still have some positive effects. Make sure to add black pepper to help the food absorb better.

Drink a cup each day

Turmeric is about the big picture approach. Consuming between 1/2 and 1/2 tsp. After four to eight weeks, the benefits of taking a daily dose of turmeric ought to become apparent.

Chili peppers for soreness and pain this active ingredient of chili peppers has been used in folk medicine for a long time and is slowly being accepted outside of homeopathy. Capsaicin is now a well-liked ingredient for topical pain relief. It works by making a certain area of the skin hot before making it numb.

Qutenza, a prescription-only capsaicin patch that relies on a very high level of capsaicin (8%), is available today.

So, what do you do if you have some cayenne pepper or hot peppers on hand and you have sore muscles or generalized body pain that won't go away? Make some cream with capsaicin.

Capsaicin coconut oil cream: Mix 3 tbsp. of coconut with one cup of cayenne powder.

- The oil should be melted when heated to a low simmer.
- For five minutes, thoroughly stir the mixture.
- Pour into a bowl after turning off the heat. Allow it to harden.
- After cooling, massage onto the skin.

Before using too much of the compound, it's important to test your reaction. You can also use jalapeo peppers, but the amount of heat they provide will vary from one pepper to the next. Wear gloves when applying this cream, and never use it on the face or around the eyes.

When you have a cold, sore throat, or are experiencing morning sickness and nausea, you should almost always try ginger. Making a cup is fairly straightforward: For a more potent effect, grate it and add it to your tea. However, the effectiveness of ginger as an anti-inflammatory is another benefit that goes unnoticed.

Try ginger the next time you feel uneasy or have a headache. Ginger has a different effect than other anti-inflammatory pain relievers. Through an antioxidant that interacts with the acidity in the fluid between the joints, it prevents the formation of certain types of inflammatory compounds and breaks down existing inflammation. No steroidal anti-inflammatory drugs (NSAIDs) carry the potential side effects associated with their anti-inflammatory effects.

- Recipe for ginger tea Grate a half-inch of raw ginger.
- Pour ginger into two cups of boiling water.
- Allow to sit for five to ten minutes.
- To taste, add lemon juice and honey or agave nectar.

Lentinan, also known as AHCC or active hexose correlated compound, is an extract of shiitake mushrooms. Shiitake mushrooms for the long game At the cellular level, it encourages antioxidant and anti-inflammatory effects.

AHCC's interaction with the immune system may aid in the fight against cancer by strengthening immune systems that have been weakened by chemotherapy, according to a Petri dish study.

The next time you make bone broth, add some chopped shiitake mushrooms if you find it comforting. After four weeks, one study found that consuming 5-10 grams of shiitake mushrooms daily helped boost human immune systems.

symptoms of irritable bowel syndrome (IBS).

According to research, it helps alleviate IBS-related spasms, diarrhea, and abdominal pain alongside fiber. Peppermint reduces inflammatory pain in the digestive tract by activating an anti-pain channel in the colon. This probably explains why it works so well to treat IBS.

A peppermint oil capsule or tea may help with headaches, colds, and other body discomforts in addition to issues with digestion and the stomach.

Fenugreek for breastfeeding the seeds of fenugreek are frequently used in Asian and Mediterranean cuisine. However, this spice, which is similar to cloves, also has a number of medicinal applications.

Fenugreek can assist breastfeeding mothers in producing more milk when brewed into a tea. Fenugreek is a great water-soluble fiber that can help firm up stools for people who are having diarrhea. These seeds should absolutely be avoided if you suffer from constipation.

Fenugreek has also been found to lower blood sugar, making it a popular diabetes aid as a supplement. This is in part because fenugreek has a lot of fiber, which can help make insulin work better.

Cooking with fenugreek Ground fenugreek is frequently used in curries, dry rubs, and teas. Sprinkle it on salads or sprinkle it on yogurt for a subtle savory flavor.

Everything can benefit from magnesium-rich foods. Having muscle pain? Fatigue? More attacks with migraine? Are you

fish like salmon, mackerel, and halibut; and bananas. Proper use of home remedies is important even though most of these natural remedies don't cause much harm if taken in large quantities.

Talk to your doctor before consuming these foods on a regular basis if you are taking any medications or have a condition that is affected by your diet. Some people may also be more sensitive to dosage amounts. And if any home remedy causes an allergic reaction or makes your symptoms worse, see a doctor right away.

Keep in mind that you might not always find home remedies to be safe and effective for you. Despite the fact that these are supported by scientific studies, a single study or clinical trial may not always include a wide range of individuals or groups. What the research says is good might not always work for you.

Many of the aforementioned remedies are ones that our families have handed down to us as children and taught us, and we look forward to using them whenever we need comfort.

CHAPTER 2

TOP 6 BENEFITS OF TAKING COLLAGEN EVERYONE SHOULD BE AWARE OF THE FOLLOWING:

Pomegranate juice is beneficial for those with low blood pressure and good for the heart when consumed daily.

Chewing a few tulsi (Basil) leaves following a meal is one natural remedy for acidity. In addition to serving as an antacid because it assists the body in absorbing food, this also prevents reflux and ulcer formation.

After eating, chewing on a clove helps to lower acidity levels.

Many stomach and gastric issues can be resolved by swallowing a garlic flake with water every morning on an empty stomach.

Juice made from watermelons can relieve a headache brought on by the heat of the summer. One glass every day does wonders!

One can alleviate migraine pain by eating an apple in the morning on an empty stomach. For the next few mornings, this must be done. For the past ten years, I've been taking medication for migraines; this one has been the most effective for me.

Open six dates and boil them for 25 minutes over low heat in 1/2 liter milk. Consume three cups daily. This is the best treatment for dry cough.

Combine equal amounts of ginger juice and two teaspoons of honey. The mixture relieves the common cold, cough, and sore throat by expectorating mucus.

If you suffer from persistent indigestion or constipation, consume half a cup of cooked beets before breakfast.

Homemade Ayurvedic cough syrup. Six medium onions are peeled and chopped. The pieces should be placed in a container with four tablespoons of honey. Cover and leave them in a water shower over low intensity for two hours. Take one tablespoon every three hours after straining.

Acne and blackheads can be effectively treated with a fifteen-minute application of grated cucumber to the face, eyes, and neck.

A straightforward treatment for anemia or iron deficiency is to pound three to four soft dates with milk and a little ghee. Consuming this combination will aid in preventing anemia.

One of the most effective home remedies for reducing dark circles is tomato paste. It is simple to make at home. Take one or two fresh tomatoes, one tablespoon of lemon juice, a pinch each of gram flour and turmeric powder, and mix them all together. Apply the mixture gently around your eyes after thoroughly blending it into a thick paste. After ten to twenty minutes, gently rinse it off with clean water. If you do this twice or three times a week, your skin around your eyes will get lighter and your dark circles will eventually disappear completely.

Gargle with salt and turmeric for the best natural treatment for a sore throat. Mix: 12 cup warm water, 1/2 teaspoon salt, and 1/4 teaspoon powdered turmeric are all you need to make a gargle. Wait at least 12 hours before drinking or eating anything to allow the salt and turmeric to kill bacteria. This can be done as many times as you need to throughout the day.

An ear infection can be helped by rubbing garlic juice into your ear.

CHAPTER 3

BODY ODOR CAN BE REDUCED BY APPLYING BAKING SODA AND LEMON JUICE TO THE UNDERARMS.

Baking soda and lemons make a natural cleaner. Put a few fennel seeds in some hot water and bring it to a low boil for five minutes. Drink the solution after straining it. If you can handle the taste, you can also chew the fresh plants with the leaves of fennel. Alternately, you can boil fennel, cardamom, and mint leaves in water to make a beverage that can alleviate gas in the stomach.

Lemon is one of the world's richest sources of vitamin C, and it also contains nutrients like vitamin B, riboflavin, phosphorus, magnesium, and calcium. This is a very effective home remedy for gas and bloating. You can also use lemon juice as a liver tonic and help eliminate waste from your system by mixing it with warm water. Lemon water consumption has a number of health benefits: It safeguards your digestive system; acts as a treatment for indigestion, high blood pressure, stress, depression, heartburn, and nausea.

A banana milkshake topped with honey can do wonders for a hangover sufferer. The lining of the stomach is soothed by cold milk, and bananas with honey replenish low blood sugar levels.

Home Remedies for a Cough: Mix honey, garlic juice, and tulsi juice to treat a severe cough. This mixture treats excessive coughing when taken once every three hours.

Natural cures for common ailments Van Sloun_Nancy_60 Nancy Van Sloun, MD Posted November 28, 2015 I wish that being a doctor would guarantee that neither my family nor I would ever become ill. Sadly, illnesses caused by viruses, bacteria, and other sources do not discriminate based on occupation. This is what's in my tool compartment to move us along in disorder and in wellbeing.

Tea - teas with fixings like licorice and tricky elm have throat-covering properties that assist with diminishing aggravation.

Honey can alleviate coughing and soothe sore throats thanks to its ability to coat the throat. Take a spoonful or mix it into your tea.

When taken within the first day or two of a cold, echinacea* can shorten the duration of symptoms. It comes in tea, drops, and pills.

Elderberry syrup* is beneficial for influenza and colds due to its antiviral properties. Follow the instructions on the package.

Pelargonium* is a plant that is used to treat coughs and colds naturally. It reduces the severity and duration of colds.

*Try each one separately to see which one you like best; Avoid using all three at once.

Have you run out of home remedies? Start a search on the internet for digestive home remedies Ginger is helpful for nausea, motion sickness, and upset stomachs. Available in the form of a tea (look for medicinal brands) or candied ginger for on-the-go consumption.

Probiotics are live strains of beneficial bacteria and yeast for the digestive system. Infection-related or antibiotic-related diarrhea can be alleviated with probiotics. Consumable in yogurt, miso paste, kombucha, kimchi, and raw sauerkraut, as well as in supplements.

Products for soreness and irritation of the skin Arnica cream treats bruises and aches in the muscles.

Tea tree oil is an anti-inflammatory treatment for infections caused by fungi or bacteria. It can be used to treat athlete's foot and acne spots.

Tea: Try drinking chamomile tea in the evening as you wind down for sleep.

Lavender is relaxing and calming aromatherapy oil. Safe for adults and young children alike.

Natural ways to deal with anxiety before you start your day, take five minutes to breathe slowly and deeply. Learn your children to use breathing exercises on the way to school to help them prepare for the day ahead. While you are there, think about the day ahead, the things you are grateful for, and the people in your life. By inhaling for four seconds and exhaling for six seconds, you can slow down your breathing. The part of the nervous system that helps us relax is triggered by this.

You can listen to calming music on your way to work or school.

Prepare for the transition home for a few minutes after work. Put the unresolved issues at work behind you and concentrate on your family.

A note on security: Inform your physician of any herbal supplements or treatments you are taking. If you are pregnant, breastfeeding, or taking prescription medications, you should talk to your doctor before taking herbal supplements.

THE END